THE PREHAB ADVANTAGE

Your Surgery Logbook and Journal

Copyright © 2025 by Michael P Hogan

Paperback ISBN:

All rights reserved. No part of this publication, either writing or images, may be reproduced, distributed, or transmitted in any form or by any means, including photocopying, recording, or other electronic or mechanical methods, without the prior written permission of the publisher, except in the case of brief quotations embodied in critical reviews and certain other noncommercial uses permitted by copyright law.

All attempts have been made to verify the information contained in this book The Prehab Advantage: Your Surgery Logbook and Journal, but the author and publisher do not bear any responsibility for errors or omissions. Any perceived negative connotation of any individual, group, or company is purely unintentional. The publisher and the author strongly recommend that you consult with your physician before beginning any exercise program. You should understand that when participating in any exercise or exercise program, there is the possibility of physical injury. If you engage in this exercise or exercise program, you agree that you do so at your own risk, are voluntarily participating in these activities, assume all risk of injury to yourself, and agree to release and discharge the publisher and the author from any and all claims or causes of action, known or unknown, arising out of the contents of this book.

The publisher and the author advise you to take full responsibility for your safety and know your limits. Before practicing the skills described in this book, be sure that your equipment is well maintained and do not take risks beyond your level of experience, aptitude, training, and comfort level.

Any resemblance to places, events, or people is purely coincidental.

Published by Light Handle Press © 2025

Foreword

As a companion to *The Prehab Advantage: A Surgeon's Guide to Preparing You for Safer Surgery and Faster Recovery,* I hope this book serves both to organize and motivate you towards being ready for your day in the operating room.

The first page is your starting line – The Prehab Home Page. It's a picture of your current health and fitness and establishes the goals of our Prehab journey. Fill out the information as completely as you can. If you have access to a prehabilitation clinic, the staff will measure your distance walked in the 6-minute walk test and your grip strength at the beginning of the program. This can be measured again just before surgery to give you an indication of how far you have come. These numbers are fantastic information to have on record and should be a visual reminder of where you started, and more importantly be clear evidence of how much stronger your body gets as the surgery date grows near. If you don't have access to a prehabilitation clinic and still want this valuable information, don't worry! We can get these numbers by doing these tests at home. There is good evidence to say that a smartphone app can accurately measure your 6-minute walk distance[1], and a basic grip strength tester is available on Amazon or at your local fitness shop for less than $30 (pick it up when you are buying your resistance bands!).

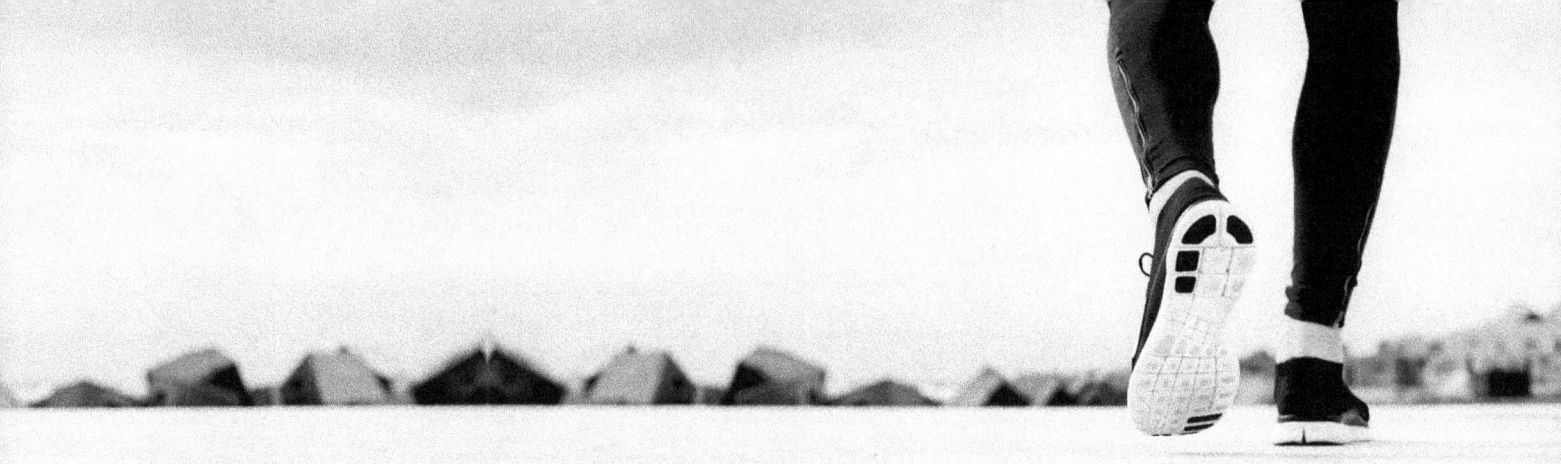

Easy Guide to Doing a 6-Minute Walk Test at Home

Before You Start

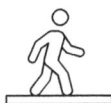 Choose a safe walking area: A flat, straight path at least 10-15 meters long (hallway, driveway, quiet street, or around your yard).

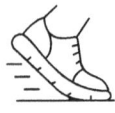 Wear comfortable shoes and loose clothing.

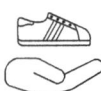 Download a 6-minute walk test app for your smartphone or get a timer (watch, phone, or stopwatch).

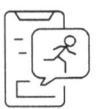 Optional but helpful: a helper to record numbers and provide support if needed.

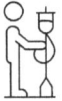 If you use a cane, walker, or portable oxygen, use them during the test.

 **Safety First**
If you feel chest pain, severe shortness of breath, dizziness, or your doctor advised against it, stop immediately.

Step-by-Step Instructions

1. **Rest before starting**
   - Sit quietly for 5 minutes. Record your resting heart rate, oxygen (if you have a pulse oximeter), and how breathless you feel.

2. **Set up the walking path**
   - Mark the starting point and measure the length of your walking course. If short, you'll walk back and forth.

3. **Start the timer**
   - Begin walking at your usual pace—fast enough to cover ground but still safe and steady.

4. **Walk continuously for 6 minutes**
   - You may slow down or stop if you need to, but restart as soon as you are able.
   - Do not run or jog.
   - Keep track of how many laps or lengths you complete.

5. **At 6 minutes**
   - Stop when the timer rings, even if you are mid-lap. Record your final position.

6. **After the test**
   - Sit down and rest.
   - Record your distance walked (laps × length + partial distance) or just look at the distance your smartphone app has recorded.
   - Record your ending heart rate, oxygen (if measured), and breathlessness.

Recording Your Results

- Total distance walked in 6 minutes (main result).
- Any symptoms (shortness of breath, fatigue, dizziness, chest discomfort).
- Rest vs. post-walk vitals (if measured).

When to Stop Immediately

- Chest pain or tightness
- Severe shortness of breath not improving with rest
- Dizziness or feeling faint
- Leg pain severe enough to stop

Smartphone Apps Can Help With

- 6-minute walk test
- Calculating your body mass index (BMI)
- Protein tracking in foods
- Exercise demonstration
- Mindful meditation

Perhaps the most important part of the front page of this journal is the section for your goals for your Prehab journey. In *The Prehab Advantage*, I outlined a basic goal template for diet, exercise, and quitting bad habits. Use these as a guide, but alter them as needed according to your age, fitness, budget, and support system. The program is difficult, and you may not reach your goals every day – but that's OK. There is no failure in Prehab. Whatever you can do will make a difference. Just remember, this is a short period of your life but could be one of the most impactful for your overall health and well-being. It's important to have a clear vision of what you want to accomplish during prehab to get your body and mind prepared for the fight ahead. By accomplishing our prehab goals, there is excellent evidence to say we can reduce our chances of complications, shorten our hospital stay, and improve our odds for a faster, complete recovery. I can't think of anything more important than that.

In addition to the physical goals you establish, be mindful of the mental battle ahead. Surgery can be a psychological roller coaster filled with emotions. As I outlined in *The Prehab Advantage*, try to spend time now to reduce the inevitable anxiety you will feel around the surgery. Part of your goal setting should include some mental preparation such as educating yourself about the process ahead or doing some mindful meditation – even if it sounds silly now, I promise it will pay off in the long run.

After the front page, this workbook starts the countdown! Prehab is typically a 4-week program prior to your surgery so the countdown will start at day 28 and go all the way to Surgery Eve. Record your daily accomplishments with diet and exercise aiming to reach your goals. If you like to journal, there is daily space for any thoughts to be jotted down. This could be anything from what protein supplements taste awful to your deepest fears about anesthesia. It will be an interesting exercise to look back on the prehab journey after it is done and review what was going through your mind as the process unfolded. These thoughts and feelings may also help to share with friends or family needing surgery in the future. Recording your experience could help others in a concrete way!

As you go through the Prehab program and put some thought into the surgery ahead, there will inevitably be questions that come up or things you don't understand about the surgery or anesthesia. Through my career, patients frequently tell me they have had questions but forget them in the heat of the moment when I'm in front of them. I've added space for you to write down any questions as you go. It's located near the back of the book – perfectly located for when the countdown is done, and you meet your team just before surgery.

The last entry for your journal will be the outcome of your surgery. Record your time in hospital, any complications you experienced, your discharge weight, and maybe even your grip strength at discharge. It will be interesting to see the effect surgery had on your body and will motivate you to get back to the fitness level you had before the operation. Finally, there will be space for a final journal entry on the whole experience.

This workbook will serve as a record of what you are capable of to optimize your body and mind for surgery, but it also has an added bonus. It is a record of what you are capable of maintaining for long-term health and well-being. It serves as documented proof that you can live an active, healthy, goal-oriented lifestyle. Grip it tightly, and use it as a springboard for a newer, healthier version of you – going through surgery might be the best thing to ever happen to your quality and quantity of life!

Good Luck and Start Prehabbing!

[1] Brooks, Gabriel C., Eric Vittinghoff, Sivaraman Iyer, Damini Tandon, Peter Kuhar, Kristine A. Madsen, Gregory M. Marcus, Mark J. Pletcher, and Jeffrey E. Olgin. 2015. "Accuracy and Usability of a Self-Administered 6-Minute Walk Test Smartphone Application." *Circulation: Heart Failure* 8 (5): 905–13.

🏠 Prehab Home Page

Name:

Phone Number: Email:

Name of Operation:

Surgery Date: Prehab Sponsor:

Phone Number:

Medical Problems:

Prior Surgery:

Medications:

Allergies:

Advanced Health Care Directive   ☐ Yes   ☐ No

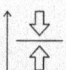 # Baseline Initial Measurements

Height:

Weight:

Body Mass Index (BMI):

6-Minute Walk Test Distance:

Grip Strength:

Cigarettes Per Day:

Alcoholic Drinks Per Day:

What is ONE Alcoholic drink
- 12 fl oz of beer
- 5 fl oz of wine
- 1.5 fl oz of liquor

 # Goals

Protein Intake: (grams per day)

Exercise: (minutes per day)

Exercise: (days per week)

Smoking: (cigarettes per day)

Drinking: (alcohol drinks per day)

Remember

For prehab we aim for about 1.5 grams of protein intake per kilogram of your weight every day

Aim to exercise 5 times a week!

Any mental health goals?

 # Other Personal Goals/Thoughts

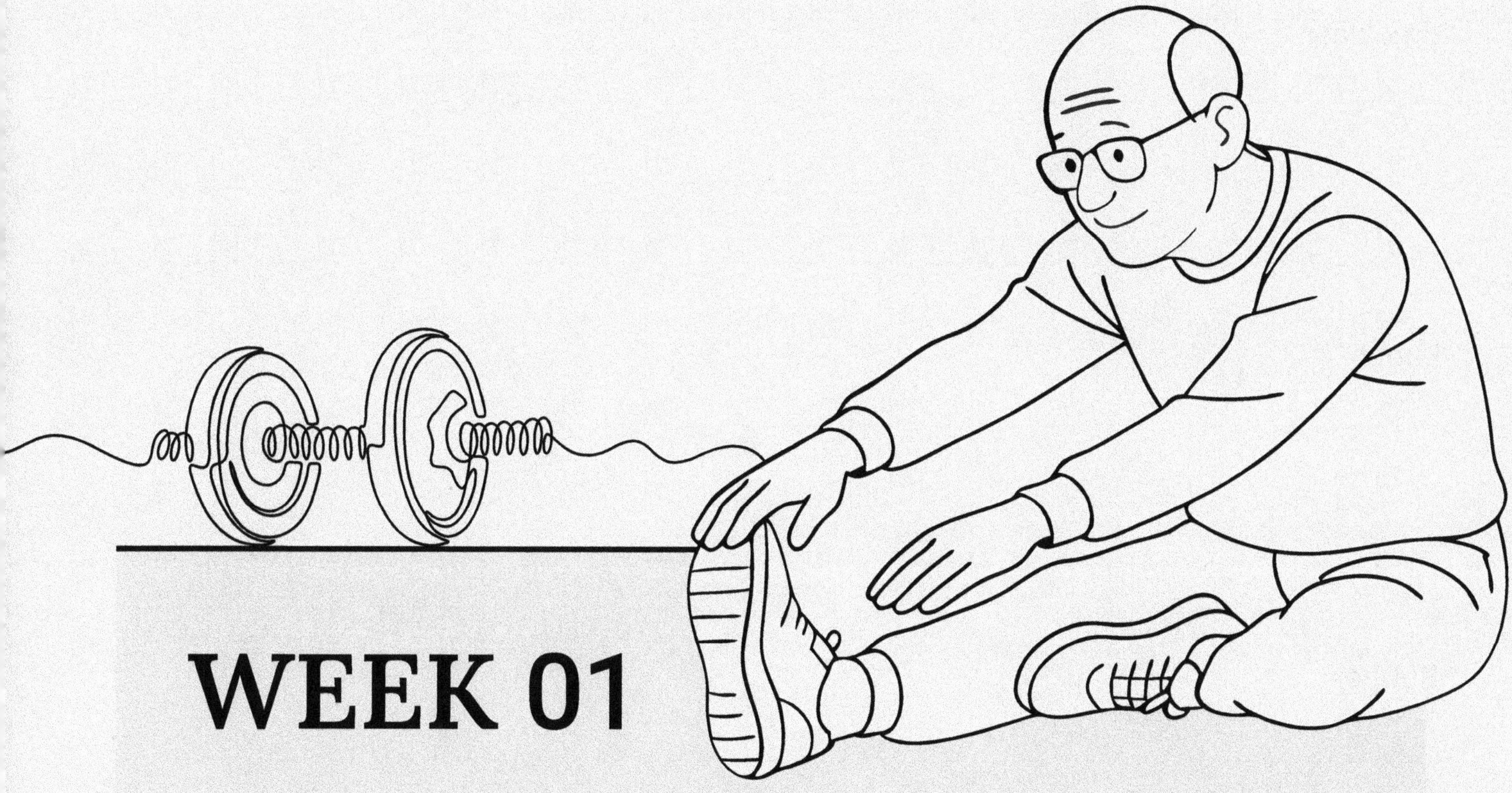

WEEK 01

 **Helpful Tips**

○ Stretch before you exercise!

○ Establish your daily routine

○ Focus on low intensity exercise this week to get started

○ Find a protein shake you like

28 Days to Surgery

Diet

Meal	What I Ate	Grams of Protein
Breakfast		
Lunch		
Supper		
Snack 1		
Snack 2		

Protein Intake Today: _____ Multivitamin Taken: _____

28 Days to Surgery

Exercise

Endurance (Aerobic)

Activity:

Time: Distance:

Reminder
Small Steps in Prehab Lead to Giant Leaps in Recovery! Any is Better Than None!

Flexibility and Stretching

Hamstring Stretch:

Hip Flexor Stretch:

Quadriceps Stretch:

Chest Stretch:

Shoulder Circles:

Stability and Posture

Pelvic tilts:

Side Planks:

Dead Bugs:

Shoulders Back/Good Posture:

Strength Training

Legs				Upper Body				Core			
Exercise	Weight	Sets	Reps	Exercise	Weight	Sets	Reps	Exercise	Weight	Sets	Reps

Journal Entry/Notes

27 Days to Surgery

🍎 Diet

Meal	What I Ate	Grams of Protein
Breakfast		
Lunch		
Supper		
Snack 1		
Snack 2		

 Protein Intake Today:  Multivitamin Taken:

27 Days to Surgery

Exercise

Endurance (Aerobic)

Activity:

Time: Distance:

Reminder
Small Steps in Prehab Lead to Giant Leaps in Recovery! Any is Better Than None!

Flexibility and Stretching

Hamstring Stretch:

Hip Flexor Stretch:

Quadriceps Stretch:

Chest Stretch:

Shoulder Circles:

Stability and Posture

Pelvic tilts:

Side Planks:

Dead Bugs:

Shoulders Back/Good Posture:

Strength Training

Legs				Upper Body				Core			
Exercise	Weight	Sets	Reps	Exercise	Weight	Sets	Reps	Exercise	Weight	Sets	Reps

Journal Entry/Notes

26 Days to Surgery

🍎 Diet

Meal	What I Ate	Grams of Protein
Breakfast		
Lunch		
Supper		
Snack 1		
Snack 2		

Protein Intake Today:  Multivitamin Taken:

26 Days to Surgery

Exercise

Endurance (Aerobic)

Activity:

Time: Distance:

Reminder
Small Steps in Prehab Lead to Giant Leaps in Recovery! Any is Better Than None!

Flexibility and Stretching

Hamstring Stretch:

Hip Flexor Stretch:

Quadriceps Stretch:

Chest Stretch:

Shoulder Circles:

Stability and Posture

Pelvic tilts:

Side Planks:

Dead Bugs:

Shoulders Back/Good Posture:

Strength Training

Legs				Upper Body				Core			
Exercise	Weight	Sets	Reps	Exercise	Weight	Sets	Reps	Exercise	Weight	Sets	Reps

Journal Entry/Notes

25 Days to Surgery

🍎 Diet

Meal	What I Ate	Grams of Protein
Breakfast		
Lunch		
Supper		
Snack 1		
Snack 2		

 Protein Intake Today:

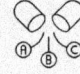 Multivitamin Taken:

25 Days to Surgery

Exercise

Endurance (Aerobic)

Activity:

Time: Distance:

Reminder
Small Steps in Prehab Lead to Giant Leaps in Recovery! Any is Better Than None!

Flexibility and Stretching

Hamstring Stretch:

Hip Flexor Stretch:

Quadriceps Stretch:

Chest Stretch:

Shoulder Circles:

Stability and Posture

Pelvic tilts:

Side Planks:

Dead Bugs:

Shoulders Back/Good Posture:

Strength Training

Legs				Upper Body				Core			
Exercise	Weight	Sets	Reps	Exercise	Weight	Sets	Reps	Exercise	Weight	Sets	Reps

Journal Entry/Notes

The Prehab Advantage | 19

24 Days to Surgery

🍎 Diet

Meal	What I Ate	Grams of Protein
Breakfast		
Lunch		
Supper		
Snack 1		
Snack 2		

Protein Intake Today:

Multivitamin Taken:

24 Days to Surgery

Exercise

Endurance (Aerobic)

Activity:

Time: Distance:

Reminder
Small Steps in Prehab Lead to Giant Leaps in Recovery! Any is Better Than None!

Flexibility and Stretching

Hamstring Stretch:

Hip Flexor Stretch:

Quadriceps Stretch:

Chest Stretch:

Shoulder Circles:

Stability and Posture

Pelvic tilts:

Side Planks:

Dead Bugs:

Shoulders Back/Good Posture:

Strength Training

Legs				Upper Body				Core			
Exercise	Weight	Sets	Reps	Exercise	Weight	Sets	Reps	Exercise	Weight	Sets	Reps

Journal Entry/Notes

The Prehab Advantage | 21

23 Days to Surgery

🍎 Diet

Meal	What I Ate	Grams of Protein
Breakfast		
Lunch		
Supper		
Snack 1		
Snack 2		

 Protein Intake Today:

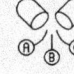 Multivitamin Taken:

23 Days to Surgery

Exercise

Endurance (Aerobic)

Activity:

Time: Distance:

Reminder
Small Steps in Prehab Lead to Giant Leaps in Recovery! Any is Better Than None!

Flexibility and Stretching

Hamstring Stretch:

Hip Flexor Stretch:

Quadriceps Stretch:

Chest Stretch:

Shoulder Circles:

Stability and Posture

Pelvic tilts:

Side Planks:

Dead Bugs:

Shoulders Back/Good Posture:

Strength Training

Legs				Upper Body				Core			
Exercise	Weight	Sets	Reps	Exercise	Weight	Sets	Reps	Exercise	Weight	Sets	Reps

Journal Entry/Notes

22 Days to Surgery

🍎 Diet

Meal	What I Ate	Grams of Protein
Breakfast		
Lunch		
Supper		
Snack 1		
Snack 2		

 Protein Intake Today: _____    Multivitamin Taken:

22 Days to Surgery

 ## Exercise

Endurance (Aerobic)

Activity:

Time: Distance:

Reminder
Small Steps in Prehab Lead to Giant Leaps in Recovery! Any is Better Than None!

Flexibility and Stretching	Stability and Posture
Hamstring Stretch:	Pelvic tilts:
Hip Flexor Stretch:	Side Planks:
Quadriceps Stretch:	Dead Bugs:
Chest Stretch:	Shoulders Back/Good Posture:
Shoulder Circles:	

Strength Training

Legs				Upper Body				Core			
Exercise	Weight	Sets	Reps	Exercise	Weight	Sets	Reps	Exercise	Weight	Sets	Reps

 ## Journal Entry/Notes

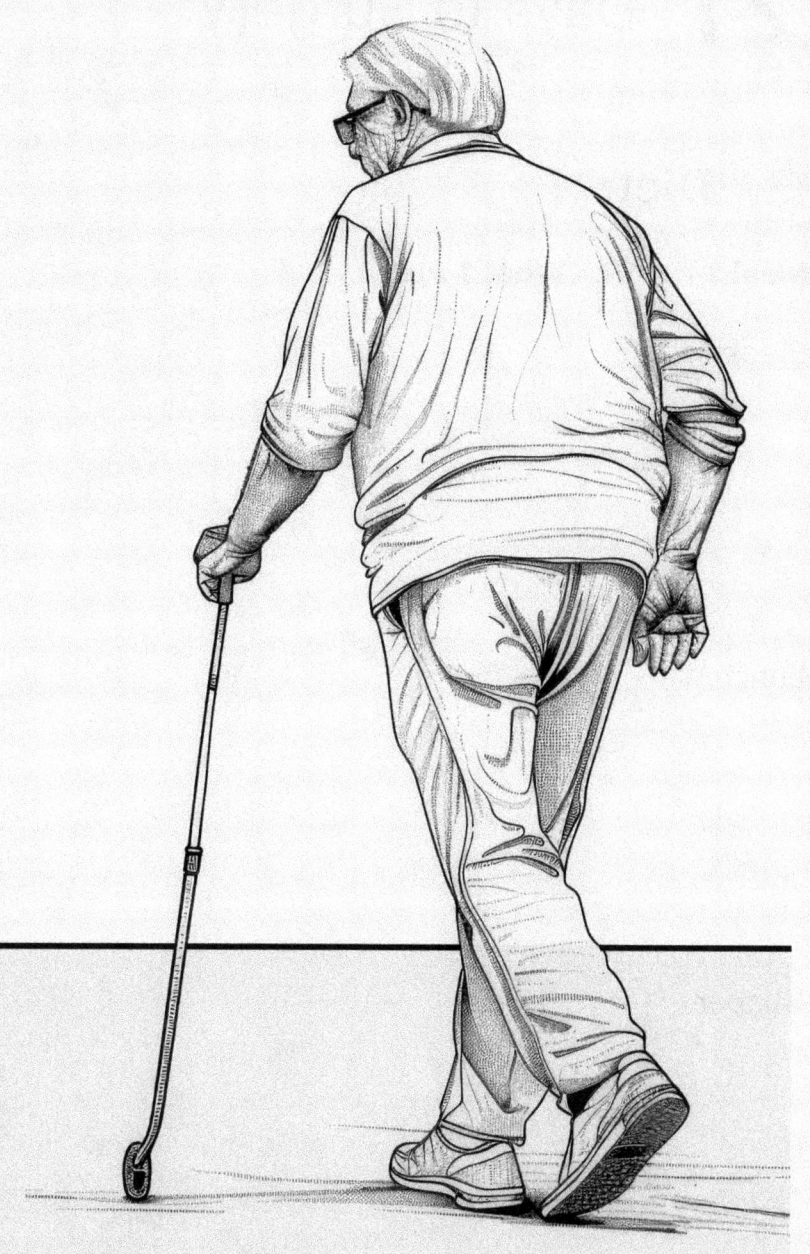

WEEK 02

 **Helpful Tips**

○ Gradually increase your exercise intensity this week

○ Aim for 20-30 minutes of walking if you can

○ Get out the resistance bands or weights for muscle building

○ Make sure you are eating enough to keep up with your activity level!

21 Days to Surgery

🍎 Diet

Meal	What I Ate	Grams of Protein
Breakfast		
Lunch		
Supper		
Snack 1		
Snack 2		

Protein Intake Today:

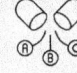 Multivitamin Taken:

21 Days to Surgery

Exercise

Endurance (Aerobic)

Activity:

Time: Distance:

Reminder
Small Steps in Prehab Lead to Giant Leaps in Recovery! Any is Better Than None!

Flexibility and Stretching

Hamstring Stretch:

Hip Flexor Stretch:

Quadriceps Stretch:

Chest Stretch:

Shoulder Circles:

Stability and Posture

Pelvic tilts:

Side Planks:

Dead Bugs:

Shoulders Back/Good Posture:

Strength Training

Legs				Upper Body				Core			
Exercise	Weight	Sets	Reps	Exercise	Weight	Sets	Reps	Exercise	Weight	Sets	Reps

Journal Entry/Notes

20 Days to Surgery

🍎 Diet

Meal	What I Ate	Grams of Protein
Breakfast		
Lunch		
Supper		
Snack 1		
Snack 2		

💪 Protein Intake Today:

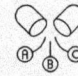 Multivitamin Taken:

20 Days to Surgery

Exercise

Endurance (Aerobic)

Activity:

Time: Distance:

Reminder
Small Steps in Prehab Lead to Giant Leaps in Recovery! Any is Better Than None!

Flexibility and Stretching

Hamstring Stretch:

Hip Flexor Stretch:

Quadriceps Stretch:

Chest Stretch:

Shoulder Circles:

Stability and Posture

Pelvic tilts:

Side Planks:

Dead Bugs:

Shoulders Back/Good Posture:

Strength Training

Legs				Upper Body				Core			
Exercise	Weight	Sets	Reps	Exercise	Weight	Sets	Reps	Exercise	Weight	Sets	Reps

Journal Entry/Notes

19 Days to Surgery

🍎 Diet

Meal	What I Ate	Grams of Protein
Breakfast		
Lunch		
Supper		
Snack 1		
Snack 2		

Protein Intake Today: _____   Multivitamin Taken:

19 Days to Surgery

Exercise

Endurance (Aerobic)

Activity:

Time: Distance:

Reminder
Small Steps in Prehab Lead to Giant Leaps in Recovery! Any is Better Than None!

Flexibility and Stretching

Hamstring Stretch:

Hip Flexor Stretch:

Quadriceps Stretch:

Chest Stretch:

Shoulder Circles:

Stability and Posture

Pelvic tilts:

Side Planks:

Dead Bugs:

Shoulders Back/Good Posture:

Strength Training

Legs				Upper Body				Core			
Exercise	Weight	Sets	Reps	Exercise	Weight	Sets	Reps	Exercise	Weight	Sets	Reps

Journal Entry/Notes

18 Days to Surgery

🍎 Diet

Meal	What I Ate	Grams of Protein
Breakfast		
Lunch		
Supper		
Snack 1		
Snack 2		

 Protein Intake Today:

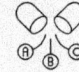 Multivitamin Taken:

18 Days to Surgery

Exercise

Endurance (Aerobic)

Activity:

Time: Distance:

Reminder
Small Steps in Prehab Lead to Giant Leaps in Recovery! Any is Better Than None!

Flexibility and Stretching

Hamstring Stretch:

Hip Flexor Stretch:

Quadriceps Stretch:

Chest Stretch:

Shoulder Circles:

Stability and Posture

Pelvic tilts:

Side Planks:

Dead Bugs:

Shoulders Back/Good Posture:

Strength Training

Legs				Upper Body				Core			
Exercise	Weight	Sets	Reps	Exercise	Weight	Sets	Reps	Exercise	Weight	Sets	Reps

Journal Entry/Notes

17 Days to Surgery

🍎 Diet

Meal	What I Ate	Grams of Protein
Breakfast		
Lunch		
Supper		
Snack 1		
Snack 2		

 Protein Intake Today:

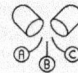 Multivitamin Taken:

17 Days to Surgery

Exercise

Endurance (Aerobic)

Activity:

Time: Distance:

Reminder
Small Steps in Prehab Lead to Giant Leaps in Recovery! Any is Better Than None!

Flexibility and Stretching

Hamstring Stretch:

Hip Flexor Stretch:

Quadriceps Stretch:

Chest Stretch:

Shoulder Circles:

Stability and Posture

Pelvic tilts:

Side Planks:

Dead Bugs:

Shoulders Back/Good Posture:

Strength Training

Legs				Upper Body				Core			
Exercise	Weight	Sets	Reps	Exercise	Weight	Sets	Reps	Exercise	Weight	Sets	Reps

Journal Entry/Notes

16 Days to Surgery

🍎 Diet

Meal	What I Ate	Grams of Protein
Breakfast		
Lunch		
Supper		
Snack 1		
Snack 2		

 Protein Intake Today:  Multivitamin Taken:

16 Days to Surgery

Exercise

Endurance (Aerobic)

Activity:

Time: Distance:

Reminder
Small Steps in Prehab Lead to Giant Leaps in Recovery! Any is Better Than None!

Flexibility and Stretching

Hamstring Stretch:

Hip Flexor Stretch:

Quadriceps Stretch:

Chest Stretch:

Shoulder Circles:

Stability and Posture

Pelvic tilts:

Side Planks:

Dead Bugs:

Shoulders Back/Good Posture:

Strength Training

Legs				Upper Body				Core			
Exercise	Weight	Sets	Reps	Exercise	Weight	Sets	Reps	Exercise	Weight	Sets	Reps

Journal Entry/Notes

The Prehab Advantage

15 Days to Surgery

🍎 Diet

Meal	What I Ate	Grams of Protein
Breakfast		
Lunch		
Supper		
Snack 1		
Snack 2		

Protein Intake Today:

Multivitamin Taken:

15 Days to Surgery

 ## Exercise

Endurance (Aerobic)

Activity:

Time: Distance:

Reminder
Small Steps in Prehab Lead to Giant Leaps in Recovery! Any is Better Than None!

Flexibility and Stretching

Hamstring Stretch:

Hip Flexor Stretch:

Quadriceps Stretch:

Chest Stretch:

Shoulder Circles:

Stability and Posture

Pelvic tilts:

Side Planks:

Dead Bugs:

Shoulders Back/Good Posture:

Strength Training

Legs				Upper Body				Core			
Exercise	Weight	Sets	Reps	Exercise	Weight	Sets	Reps	Exercise	Weight	Sets	Reps

 ## Journal Entry/Notes

The Prehab Advantage | 41

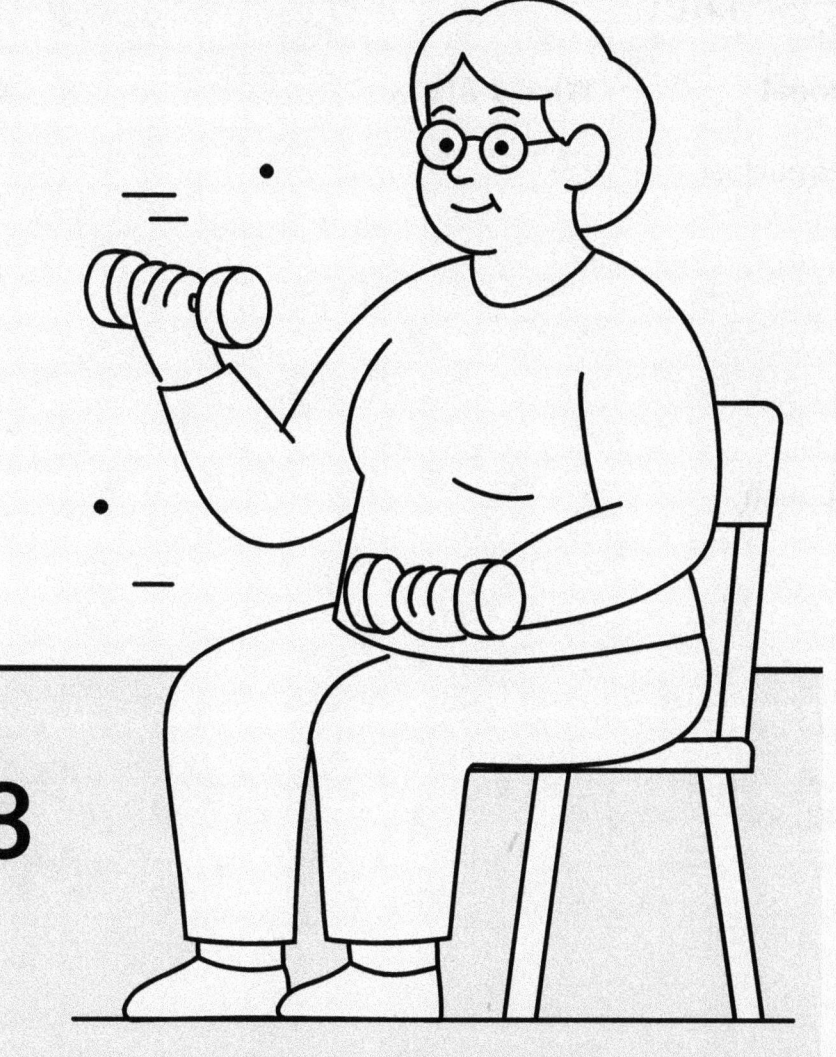

WEEK 03

 **Helpful Tips**

○ Keep at it! You are halfway there already!

○ Build on your progress and aim for a 30-minute walk at least 5 times this week

○ Increase the resistance for muscle building

○ Don't forget to spend some quiet time thinking about the progress you are making

14 Days to Surgery

🍎 Diet

Meal	What I Ate	Grams of Protein
Breakfast		
Lunch		
Supper		
Snack 1		
Snack 2		

Protein Intake Today:

Multivitamin Taken:

14 Days to Surgery

Exercise

Endurance (Aerobic)

Activity:

Time: Distance:

Reminder
Small Steps in Prehab Lead to Giant Leaps in Recovery! Any is Better Than None!

Flexibility and Stretching

Hamstring Stretch:

Hip Flexor Stretch:

Quadriceps Stretch:

Chest Stretch:

Shoulder Circles:

Stability and Posture

Pelvic tilts:

Side Planks:

Dead Bugs:

Shoulders Back/Good Posture:

Strength Training

Legs				Upper Body				Core			
Exercise	Weight	Sets	Reps	Exercise	Weight	Sets	Reps	Exercise	Weight	Sets	Reps

Journal Entry/Notes

13 Days to Surgery

🍎 Diet

Meal	What I Ate	Grams of Protein
Breakfast		
Lunch		
Supper		
Snack 1		
Snack 2		

 Protein Intake Today:  Multivitamin Taken:

13 Days to Surgery

🏃 Exercise

Endurance (Aerobic)		Reminder
Activity:		Small Steps in Prehab Lead to Giant Leaps in Recovery! Any is Better Than None!
Time:	Distance:	

Flexibility and Stretching	Stability and Posture
Hamstring Stretch:	Pelvic tilts:
Hip Flexor Stretch:	Side Planks:
Quadriceps Stretch:	Dead Bugs:
Chest Stretch:	Shoulders Back/Good Posture:
Shoulder Circles:	

🏋 Strength Training

Legs				Upper Body				Core			
Exercise	Weight	Sets	Reps	Exercise	Weight	Sets	Reps	Exercise	Weight	Sets	Reps

 Journal Entry/Notes

12 Days to Surgery

🍎 Diet

Meal	What I Ate	Grams of Protein
Breakfast		
Lunch		
Supper		
Snack 1		
Snack 2		

Protein Intake Today:

Multivitamin Taken:

12 Days to Surgery

Exercise

Endurance (Aerobic)

Activity:

Time: Distance:

Reminder
Small Steps in Prehab Lead to Giant Leaps in Recovery! Any is Better Than None!

Flexibility and Stretching

Hamstring Stretch:

Hip Flexor Stretch:

Quadriceps Stretch:

Chest Stretch:

Shoulder Circles:

Stability and Posture

Pelvic tilts:

Side Planks:

Dead Bugs:

Shoulders Back/Good Posture:

Strength Training

Legs				Upper Body				Core			
Exercise	Weight	Sets	Reps	Exercise	Weight	Sets	Reps	Exercise	Weight	Sets	Reps

Journal Entry/Notes

The Prehab Advantage | 49

11 Days to Surgery

🍎 Diet

Meal	What I Ate	Grams of Protein
Breakfast		
Lunch		
Supper		
Snack 1		
Snack 2		

 Protein Intake Today:

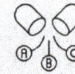 Multivitamin Taken:

11 Days to Surgery

Exercise

Endurance (Aerobic)

Activity:

Time: Distance:

Reminder
Small Steps in Prehab Lead to Giant Leaps in Recovery! Any is Better Than None!

Flexibility and Stretching

Hamstring Stretch:

Hip Flexor Stretch:

Quadriceps Stretch:

Chest Stretch:

Shoulder Circles:

Stability and Posture

Pelvic tilts:

Side Planks:

Dead Bugs:

Shoulders Back/Good Posture:

Strength Training

Legs				Upper Body				Core			
Exercise	Weight	Sets	Reps	Exercise	Weight	Sets	Reps	Exercise	Weight	Sets	Reps

Journal Entry/Notes

10 Days to Surgery

🍎 Diet

Meal	What I Ate	Grams of Protein
Breakfast		
Lunch		
Supper		
Snack 1		
Snack 2		

 Protein Intake Today: _____    Multivitamin Taken: _____

10 Days to Surgery

Exercise

Endurance (Aerobic)

Activity:

Time: Distance:

Reminder
Small Steps in Prehab Lead to Giant Leaps in Recovery! Any is Better Than None!

Flexibility and Stretching

Hamstring Stretch:

Hip Flexor Stretch:

Quadriceps Stretch:

Chest Stretch:

Shoulder Circles:

Stability and Posture

Pelvic tilts:

Side Planks:

Dead Bugs:

Shoulders Back/Good Posture:

Strength Training

Legs				Upper Body				Core			
Exercise	Weight	Sets	Reps	Exercise	Weight	Sets	Reps	Exercise	Weight	Sets	Reps

Journal Entry/Notes

The Prehab Advantage | 53

9 Days to Surgery

🍎 Diet

Meal	What I Ate	Grams of Protein
Breakfast		
Lunch		
Supper		
Snack 1		
Snack 2		

 Protein Intake Today:  Multivitamin Taken:

9 Days to Surgery

Exercise

Endurance (Aerobic)

Activity:

Time: Distance:

Reminder
Small Steps in Prehab Lead to Giant Leaps in Recovery! Any is Better Than None!

Flexibility and Stretching

Hamstring Stretch:

Hip Flexor Stretch:

Quadriceps Stretch:

Chest Stretch:

Shoulder Circles:

Stability and Posture

Pelvic tilts:

Side Planks:

Dead Bugs:

Shoulders Back/Good Posture:

Strength Training

Legs				Upper Body				Core			
Exercise	Weight	Sets	Reps	Exercise	Weight	Sets	Reps	Exercise	Weight	Sets	Reps

Journal Entry/Notes

The Prehab Advantage | 55

8 Days to Surgery

🍎 Diet

Meal	What I Ate	Grams of Protein
Breakfast		
Lunch		
Supper		
Snack 1		
Snack 2		

 Protein Intake Today:

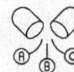 Multivitamin Taken:

8 Days to Surgery

Exercise

Endurance (Aerobic)

Activity:

Time: Distance:

Reminder
Small Steps in Prehab Lead to Giant Leaps in Recovery! Any is Better Than None!

Flexibility and Stretching

Hamstring Stretch:

Hip Flexor Stretch:

Quadriceps Stretch:

Chest Stretch:

Shoulder Circles:

Stability and Posture

Pelvic tilts:

Side Planks:

Dead Bugs:

Shoulders Back/Good Posture:

Strength Training

Legs

Exercise	Weight	Sets	Reps

Upper Body

Exercise	Weight	Sets	Reps

Core

Exercise	Weight	Sets	Reps

Journal Entry/Notes

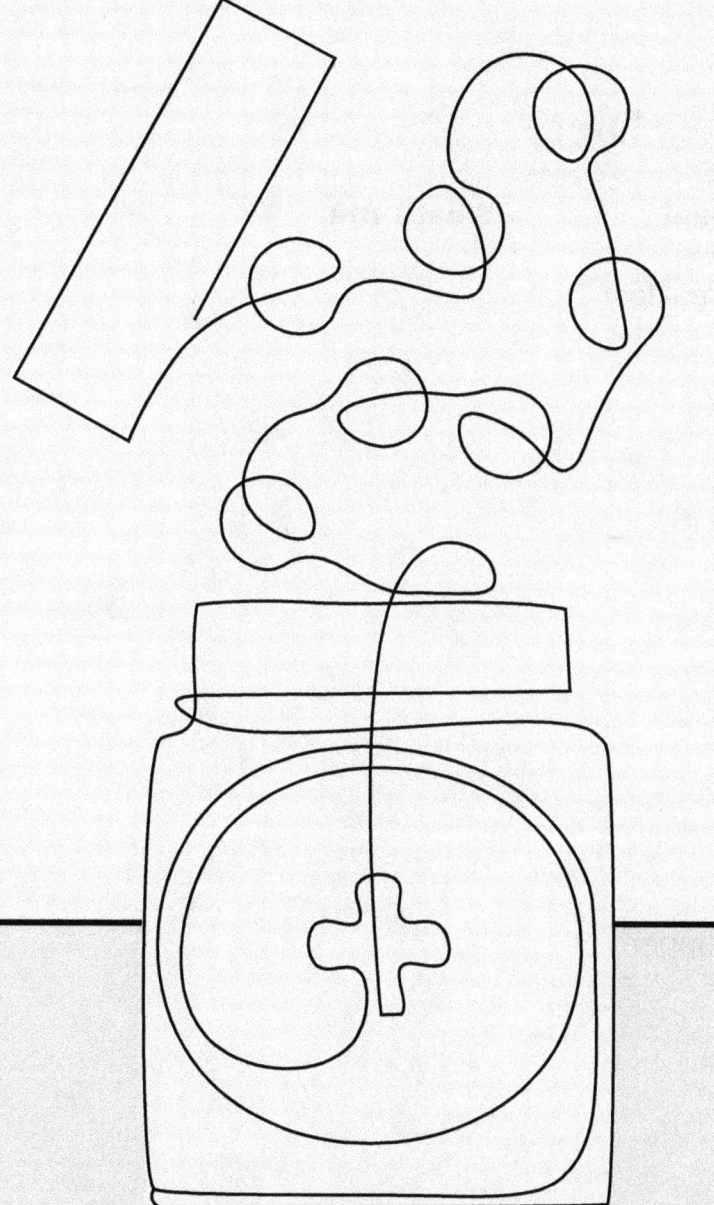

WEEK 04

 Helpful Tips

○ Final push before surgery!

○ Add immunonutrition supplements to your diet this week

○ Aim for moderate intensity across all exercises and don't forget the stretching

7 Days to Surgery

Diet

Meal	What I Ate	Grams of Protein
Breakfast		
Lunch		
Supper		
Snack 1		
Snack 2		

Protein Intake Today:

Multivitamin Taken:

7 Days to Surgery

🏃 Exercise

Endurance (Aerobic)		**Reminder**
Activity:		Small Steps in Prehab Lead to Giant Leaps in Recovery! Any is Better Than None!
Time:	Distance:	

Flexibility and Stretching	**Stability and Posture**
Hamstring Stretch:	Pelvic tilts:
Hip Flexor Stretch:	Side Planks:
Quadriceps Stretch:	Dead Bugs:
Chest Stretch:	Shoulders Back/Good Posture:
Shoulder Circles:	

🏋 Strength Training

Legs				Upper Body				Core			
Exercise	Weight	Sets	Reps	Exercise	Weight	Sets	Reps	Exercise	Weight	Sets	Reps

Journal Entry/Notes

6 Days to Surgery

🍎 Diet

Meal	What I Ate	Grams of Protein
Breakfast		
Lunch		
Supper		
Snack 1		
Snack 2		

 Protein Intake Today:

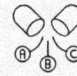 Multivitamin Taken:

6 Days to Surgery

 ## Exercise

Endurance (Aerobic)

Activity:

Time: Distance:

Reminder
Small Steps in Prehab Lead to Giant Leaps in Recovery! Any is Better Than None!

Flexibility and Stretching

Hamstring Stretch:

Hip Flexor Stretch:

Quadriceps Stretch:

Chest Stretch:

Shoulder Circles:

Stability and Posture

Pelvic tilts:

Side Planks:

Dead Bugs:

Shoulders Back/Good Posture:

Strength Training

Legs				Upper Body				Core			
Exercise	Weight	Sets	Reps	Exercise	Weight	Sets	Reps	Exercise	Weight	Sets	Reps

 ## Journal Entry/Notes

5 Days to Surgery

🍎 Diet

Meal	What I Ate	Grams of Protein
Breakfast		
Lunch		
Supper		
Snack 1		
Snack 2		

 Protein Intake Today:  Multivitamin Taken:

5 Days to Surgery

Exercise

Endurance (Aerobic)

Activity:

Time: Distance:

Reminder
Small Steps in Prehab Lead to Giant Leaps in Recovery! Any is Better Than None!

Flexibility and Stretching

Hamstring Stretch:

Hip Flexor Stretch:

Quadriceps Stretch:

Chest Stretch:

Shoulder Circles:

Stability and Posture

Pelvic tilts:

Side Planks:

Dead Bugs:

Shoulders Back/Good Posture:

Strength Training

Legs				Upper Body				Core			
Exercise	Weight	Sets	Reps	Exercise	Weight	Sets	Reps	Exercise	Weight	Sets	Reps

Journal Entry/Notes

4 Days to Surgery

🍎 Diet

Meal	What I Ate	Grams of Protein
Breakfast		
Lunch		
Supper		
Snack 1		
Snack 2		

Protein Intake Today:  Multivitamin Taken:

4 Days to Surgery

🏃 Exercise

Endurance (Aerobic)

Activity:

Time: Distance:

Reminder
Small Steps in Prehab Lead to Giant Leaps in Recovery! Any is Better Than None!

Flexibility and Stretching

Hamstring Stretch:

Hip Flexor Stretch:

Quadriceps Stretch:

Chest Stretch:

Shoulder Circles:

Stability and Posture

Pelvic tilts:

Side Planks:

Dead Bugs:

Shoulders Back/Good Posture:

🏋 Strength Training

Legs				Upper Body				Core			
Exercise	Weight	Sets	Reps	Exercise	Weight	Sets	Reps	Exercise	Weight	Sets	Reps

Journal Entry/Notes

3 Days to Surgery

🍎 Diet

Meal	What I Ate	Grams of Protein
Breakfast		
Lunch		
Supper		
Snack 1		
Snack 2		

 Protein Intake Today:

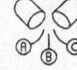 Multivitamin Taken:

3 Days to Surgery

Exercise

Endurance (Aerobic)

Activity:

Time: Distance:

Reminder
Small Steps in Prehab Lead to Giant Leaps in Recovery! Any is Better Than None!

Flexibility and Stretching

Hamstring Stretch:

Hip Flexor Stretch:

Quadriceps Stretch:

Chest Stretch:

Shoulder Circles:

Stability and Posture

Pelvic tilts:

Side Planks:

Dead Bugs:

Shoulders Back/Good Posture:

Strength Training

Legs				Upper Body				Core			
Exercise	Weight	Sets	Reps	Exercise	Weight	Sets	Reps	Exercise	Weight	Sets	Reps

Journal Entry/Notes

The Prehab Advantage | 69

2 Days to Surgery

🍎 Diet

Meal	What I Ate	Grams of Protein
Breakfast		
Lunch		
Supper		
Snack 1		
Snack 2		

 Protein Intake Today:  Multivitamin Taken:

2 Days to Surgery

🏃 Exercise

Endurance (Aerobic)		Reminder
Activity:		Small Steps in Prehab Lead to Giant Leaps in Recovery! Any is Better Than None!
Time:	Distance:	

Flexibility and Stretching	Stability and Posture
Hamstring Stretch:	Pelvic tilts:
Hip Flexor Stretch:	Side Planks:
Quadriceps Stretch:	Dead Bugs:
Chest Stretch:	Shoulders Back/Good Posture:
Shoulder Circles:	

🏋️ Strength Training

Legs				Upper Body				Core			
Exercise	Weight	Sets	Reps	Exercise	Weight	Sets	Reps	Exercise	Weight	Sets	Reps

Journal Entry/Notes

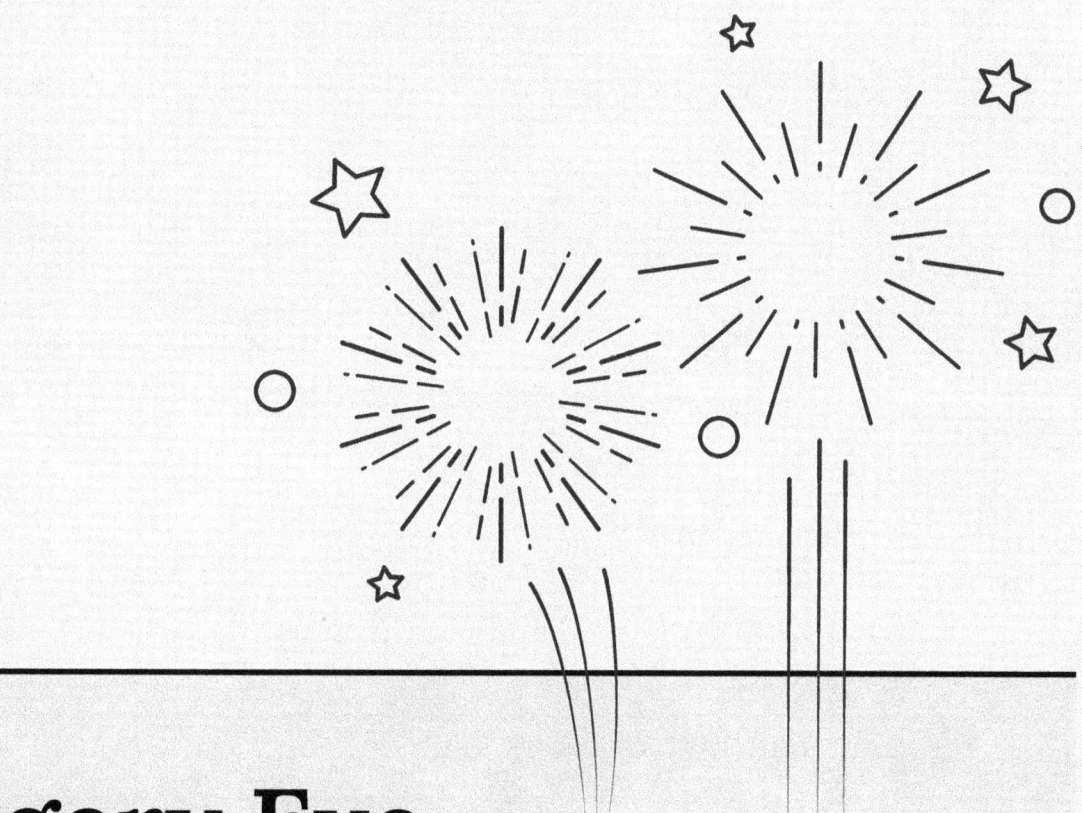

Surgery Eve

 Helpful Tips

○ Congratulations – you've graduated from Prehab! You have done everything in your power to contribute to your surgical success

○ Fill out the Post Prehab Measurements to see your progress

○ You may want to take a recovery day today from exercise
 - you've earned it

○ Follow the fasting and medication instructions provided by your hospital

○ Don't forget your carbohydrate drink two hours before surgery
 IF your hospital allows it

○ Make sure you have your questions for the team written down
 (if you have any)

1 Day to Surgery

🍎 Diet

Meal	What I Ate	Grams of Protein
Breakfast		
Lunch		
Supper		
Snack 1		
Snack 2		

 Protein Intake Today:  Multivitamin Taken:

1 Day to Surgery

🏃 Exercise

Endurance (Aerobic)

Activity:

Time: Distance:

Reminder
Small Steps in Prehab Lead to Giant Leaps in Recovery! Any is Better Than None!

Flexibility and Stretching

Hamstring Stretch:

Hip Flexor Stretch:

Quadriceps Stretch:

Chest Stretch:

Shoulder Circles:

Stability and Posture

Pelvic tilts:

Side Planks:

Dead Bugs:

Shoulders Back/Good Posture:

🏋 Strength Training

Legs				Upper Body				Core			
Exercise	Weight	Sets	Reps	Exercise	Weight	Sets	Reps	Exercise	Weight	Sets	Reps

 Journal Entry/Notes

The Prehab Advantage

Post Prehab Measurements

Height:

Weight:

Body Mass Index (BMI):

6-Minute Walk Test Distance:

Grip Strength:

Cigarettes Per Day:

Alcoholic Drinks Per Day:

What is ONE **Alcoholic drink**
- 12 fl oz of beer
- 5 fl oz of wine
- 1.5 fl oz of liquor

Reflections on Your Goals - How did you do?

Diet:

Exercise:

Mental Health:

Bad Habits:

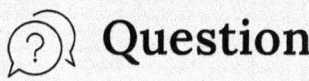
Questions

Questions for your anesthesiologist

Questions for your surgeon

My Surgery Experience

Name of Operation:

Surgeon:

Anesthesiologist:

Favorite Nurse:

Least Favorite Meal:

Time in Hospital:

Complications:

Weight at Discharge:

Grip strength at Discharge:

Impact of Prehab:

Reflections:

If you feel that Prehab had an impact on your surgery experience, write a review on Amazon so that others can benefit as well!

www.ingramcontent.com/pod-product-compliance
Lightning Source LLC
Chambersburg PA
CBHW081202020426
42333CB00020B/2605